Relax! It's Only Cancer!

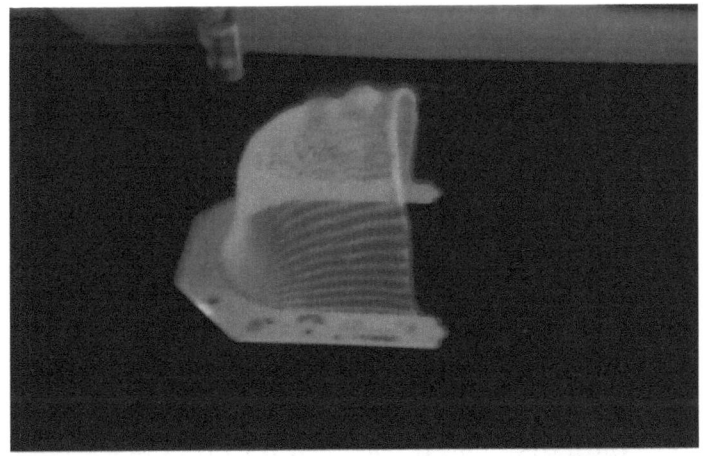

The mask commonly used to hold

patients head in the correct position during

radiation treatments; this particular mask was mine!

A practical *"how to"* book; when dealing with cancer treatments. Chemotherapy and radiation treatments are difficult experiences for cancer patients. The information in this book will ease much of the pain caused by the side effects of these treatments!

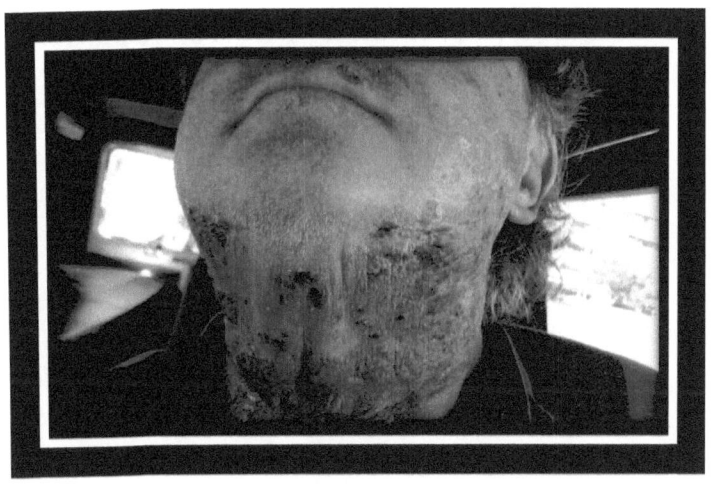

Radiation treatments had my neck looking like this before I started treating myself for the side effects; this photo was after four weeks of treatments, I was scheduled for, and completed nine weeks of treatments! Much of this pain was not necessary, but I did not know then what I know now. Although I received radiation treatments for nine weeks; the worst pictures were taken during the fourth and fifth week of treatments. That is when I started treating myself for the side effects; even though I continued receiving the treatments, my neck was completely healed by the time I finished the ninth week! The picture below was taken during week seven of treatments. Already my neck was much improved.

(PICTURE)

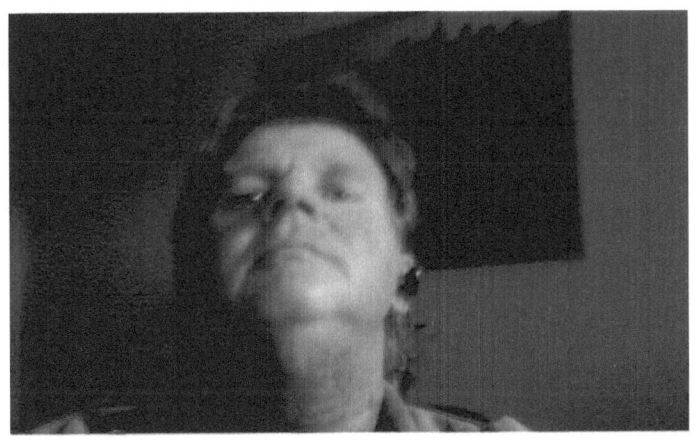

Inside this book, you will find amazing products that will make cancer patients more comfortable during the challenging days when they're receiving chemotherapy and radiation treatments.

I firmly believe, if I ever have to go through chemo and radiation again; by using the near miraculous products listed in this book from the time of the first treatment forward; I could nearly eliminate the side effects!

Contents:

Introduction:

Chapter One: Cancer Interrupts Life

Chapter Two: Cancer Funk

Chapter Three: What to Expect from Cancer Treatments

Chapter Four: That Knowing Smile

Chapter Five: Amazing Products

Chapter Six: A Toast: "Here's to Remission"

Chapter Seven: Aftermath; Continuing the Healing Process

Chapter Eight: The-- *Why Me?*—Thing

Chapter One

Cancer Interrupts Life

Four days before the scheduled date of my hip replacement surgery, during a pre-operation office visit, my doctor noticed the lymph nodes on both sides of my neck were swollen. He immediately postponed my hip replacement surgery, and instead sent me to an ear, nose and throat specialist (ENT) to see why my glands were swollen. It wasn't long before several test revealed that I had cancer of the tonsils!

I felt that cancer interrupted my life. It interfered with my future plans. It cluttered my daily schedule with doctor appointments I did not want to attend. It seemed to come into my life at the worst time; I wanted it to just go away, I told myself over and over again,

"All I have to do is change my schedule for about five months while finishing up the chemotherapy and radiation, and then just pick up my life where I had left off." That seemed so logical to me, and it was that thought and the hopes that accompanied it that kept me from feeling hopelessly depressed. I just had to put all my plans on hold until after I dealt with my cancer problem, and in my naive mind, that was exactly what I planned to do.

But when I woke up from my surgical biopsy; my doctor not only informed me that he had found three cancerous tumors in and around my tonsils; because they were attached to my collated artery and my vocal cords, he was unable to remove them completely. He had however, removed half of each of the three tumors. He also told me that the type of cancer I had was not curable! It would never go completely away; I was told I had 47% chance of living five more years, and only 18% chance of living ten more years! The air itself roared like wolves howling when my doctor told me the bad news!

 What I did not realize then is that cancer does not just interrupt our lives, it also becomes part of our lives, part of who we are and what we are all about! There is no convenient time to have cancer! Everyone feels it interrupted their schedule, but face the facts here; would a year earlier have been better for you?

Even when it is in remission; you will then be a cancer survivor; in short, there is no going back, you may regain your health and beat cancer completely and I certainly hope that is your good fortune; but re-boarding the good ship lolly-pop is out of the question, you're not in Kansas anymore! You have cancer, and the experience is usually life changing.

I was told the combination of surgery, chemotherapy, and radiation treatments would temporarily slow cancer's progress and enable me to live in a reasonability healthy state for an unknown length of time; so, I decided it was my best shot at ever being healthy again. I also began taking several herb and vitamin pills, as an alternate form of healing. (Those products are listed later in the book.)

So my plan of taking a few months treatments and then moving on with my life crumbled right before my eyes. Now, new questions were popping into my mind, questions no one could answer with any certainty; all of the questions involved cancers unknown impact on my future health. I found it difficult to make future plans. I wondered if I even had a future! I had a lot to learn.

Chapter Two

Curing Cancer Funk

While cancer was my physical enemy, pre-conceived notions were my mental enemies. I entered a state of mind I called a cancer funk. The first mental mistake I made was trying to figure out how I'd caused my cancer. Something I'd done must have caused me to get this horrid disease. But, I had never been a smoker, so perhaps it wasn't something I was directly responsible for; yet, even if it was not caused by my actions, perhaps I was somehow to blame indirectly, I wondered if I had angered God somehow, was I being punished by the supreme power of the universe? Right about then, I wondered if I would I ever be happy again. It did not make any sense to me to start a new romance, or further my education, or make long term career choices when, in reality, I may die very soon. How was I supposed to be excited or positive about making any plans for my long term future, knowing I have incurable cancer? I started to plan my own death!

Fortunately for my I have a very canny Uncle. My Uncle Don, retired from being a fire chief; gave me some words of wisdom I could really hold onto. This is what he said, "I have seen countless firemen retire and many others had to leave their chosen profession because of serious injuries; but I have noticed one common trait that every person who successfully made the necessary changes in their lives; and it is a trait that is obviously missing from those who cannot adjust to changes; here is the one trait we all must process to be successful at nearly anything in this life. *We all have to plan to keep living!*

It was as if the thought fairy had waved a magic thought wand on me! What a profound, yet simple thought. Yes I thought, it I plan on living, and I end up dying; I will just be another person who didn't finish all his plans and projects. But if I keep thinking about dying, I soon will not make any plans, and then what, just sit around waiting for the Grim Reaper? That's not for me! I soon decided I was going to live until I die, and I would have plans right up until then.

This was a big key in shaking off the cancer funk that was giving me the blues! I became quietly busy; oh, I kept it a secret, but I soon resented the cancer funk into which I had temporality fallen and I was determined to make plans to continue living; and I have done just that! I finally fought through it; I realized certain thoughts were common cancer lies, tricks that occur in the minds of many cancer victims. I set out to rid myself of cancer funk forever!

The key to learning the truth was interacting with other cancer patients. I soon was interacting with every cancer patient I found! I learned, in most instances, we were all thinking along the same lines. For me, this became a turning point.

At the time, I justified my thoughts and worries; but interacting with a large group of cancer patients on a daily basis and hearing them voice the same concerns I had; I suddenly realized the truth. Looking at the large room filled with cancer patients, I suddenly realized we were not all going to die from cancer, neither were we all going to die soon! Many of us, now fighting our first round with cancer, would win! Others may have to fight round two before they won their health back. Only a small percentage of us would die from cancer! We not only could continue making plans for the future, we each owe it to ourselves and our families to do that; continue living a full life, as long as we are alive!

Although I may be a sinner of deplorable nature, and my sins may be egregious to God himself, and perhaps that is why he was punishing mc by giving me this terrible disease; as I got to know other patients, I learned many of them were good people, normal people; and as I realized they were not being punished by God, I also realized that I wasn't either! That is just piffle! Several of them told me they felt the same way at first, but as we got to know each other during our daily treatments, we each realized that although cancer had come to each of us, we deserved to be healthy again; we eventually accepted the belief that we had not angered a deity to acquire this illness, we just chalked it up to bad luck, but we all agreed; this would test us, test our faith, our trust, our beliefs; and if we passed this test, we would come away as stronger and better people!

Cancer funk, by definition, is a depression of the soul, a sadness of the spirit; caused by believing the lies that surround cancer and all its myths. Cancer causes people to stop and ponder several 'what if' questions. This group of questions is generally negative in nature and in a short time can void a life of all laughter; don't let it happen to you. Most of the questions are along the same lines, they involve the future; your security has been threatened and the 'knee jerk' reaction many people have can be summed up by this one question; *why should I make any future plans, when I may die soon?*

Don't let unfounded fears ruin your future, fill you with uncertainty and rob you of your laughter. You survived until now in life somehow, and now you've been diagnosed with cancer, and right now, you really cannot imagine anything worse; really? It is a cancer funk mind trick. It is not the truth.

My first cancer experience happened like this. Cancer came, I kicked its but, it was a battle; but I gave it everything I had; and now, it is in remission. That is the end of my first cancer experience. It took five months out of my life and perhaps another year to heal up completely, okay I only healed up to ninety per cent of what I once was; but I can still live comfortably with the results, and I can still laugh! Although at first, I could think of nothing worse. So, I made a list of ten things that would have been worse than my first cancer experience. See if you agree with my perspective;

1. Being a prisoner of war.
2. Losing a loved one in the Twin Towers attack on 9-11.
3. Suffering a lasting paralysis injury.
4. Contracting AIDS and dying from it.
5. My children or grandchildren having cancer.
6. Getting shot and killed because I came home and surprised a robber.

7. Contracting a disease that I know will eventually disable me and kill me. i.e. (Muscular Dystrophy)
8. Having your child die from drug addiction.
9. Lasting depression
10. Being addicted to alcohol or drugs.

   I could go on and on, but you get the idea. The next time you think you've got it worse than anyone else on earth; re-read the list, life could be worse, and is for many people.

I am not saying cancer isn't serious, or that it is a wimpy disease. All I'm saying is put your back into it; make the changes you need to make, get the help you need, and fight the good fight. Avoid self-pity and *bottomless* questions. (based on fears and rumors, but instead learn all the facts available to you) These questions generate lies, lies and more lies.

Here are some undeniable truths you can hang your hat on. Each of us is going to live until we die. We will all die of one thing or another. You have a disease that kills far less than half of its victims. Even if you already have cancer, your odds of dying from something entirely different than cancer are greater than your odds of dying of cancer; (does it really matter so much how you die? I'm more concerned about how I live! Ha, ha, ha, LOL) {LOL=laugh out loud} even if you have a deadly cancer and you eventually die from it, worrying about dying will not add on minute to your life.

Laughter, on the other hand, really may add years to your life, that and owning a dog, for some reason. Ha, ha, ha, LOL. Don't stop laughing because you have cancer. Don't stop having fun either. As time passes, medical professionals are winning many battles against cancer, so is alternative medicine, which cures many patients. Treatments of every kind are much better than they once were, and will continue to improve.

There are lies, damn lies, and then there are statistics! If anyone quotes you statistics on your particular cancer and stage of development, ask them three questions about their statistics.

1. Are they only for the United States, or are the statistics worldwide. Some countries have better cancer treatment facilities than others. Many countries have no major medical plans at all. The truth is; each country should publish its own cancer statics. If you live in a country with good cancer treatment

facilities, your odds are much better than the world's statics which include the countries that have little or very archaic cancer treatment policies.

2. Are they current? Cancer statistics that are two years old are outdated! Types of cancer that killed people ten years ago are now considered curable.

3. Do the statics include patients that have sought alternative treatments, outside of the traditional medical field? Don't down play this avenue

of help. I'd be the last person to advise anyone to go against doctor's orders, but many times you can do both what the doctors recommend and take alternate medicine. I recommend taking a sample of what you intend to take to your doctor and ask him if it will conflict in any way with treatments he is recommending. Many doctors today will encourage alternative cures. My doctor recommended them for me!

The thing to remember is your body wants to be healthy and this is just a setback. You may have only one bout with cancer; or you may have more than one. Treat every round as a separate battle and follow doctor's orders. Seek alternative medicine and talk it over with your doctor to make sure it gels with the treatments he is giving you. You may need counseling, if you need it, get it. You may need to make changes in your lifestyle. Make the changes you need to make. My doctor told me to get leaner but stay strong; lean muscle being a better state for my body than being overweight, with regards to cancer (and other things.) I lost weight, quit lifting heavy weights and started working out with some boxers. (But, I didn't let them punch me, just did their routines!) Make the changes you need to make, fight the good fight, and most importantly go on with your plans and your life.

Chapter Three

What to Expect from Cancer Treatments

Let me clear one thing up right now, how tough you are or are not has nothing to do with whether or not you should use these simple products to promote your comfort during chemotherapy and radiation treatments. Look at it this way, you may be tough enough to sleep on a bed of nails but why would you? Especially if a softer bed is readily available. This is a matter of keeping you as comfortable as humanly possible. If you're into comfort, read on.

 I was prepared to be a tough guy; my own history proved I could be when I put my mind to it. At first, I was doing great at being a tough guy, at enduring it all, when reality came crashing in on me. I was sitting in the waiting room next to a woman who was not dealing so well with cancer and all the side effects of her treatments. She was definitely in a cancer funk, she felt, as did I at that time, we just had to endure the pain caused by all the side effects of the treatments. Then she said something that made me realize I needed to change my thinking.

"I'm so sick of cancer treatments; this is my third time, if my cancer comes back again, rather than go through the treatments again, I'm going to kill myself!"

I was in my second week of radiation, my throat was beginning to close, and my neck was showing burns. My mouth was dry and my tongue was killing me. What she said sent my mind whirling in thought. I started looking around at some other patients, some were being wheeled in on beds, some on wheelchairs; many whose throats had closed, had feeding tubes; as I conversed with them I soon learned six of the twenty five patients were having their second round with cancer, and one woman there was fighting round three. That was when I realized that my comfort was important during cancer treatments. If my cancer returned, these treatments would become a necessarily repetitive routine in my life. They were not something evil I had to endure; barely living through; my mindset changed entirely, instead of wanting to endure all the discomforts of the treatments like a good solider; I now declared war with each side effect of chemotherapy and radiation treatments! I became pugnacious! I decided since I have cancer and these treatments were now part of my life, I might as well make the best of things, and the best of things did not include suffering through these treatments, if I could somehow avoid it. My docile attitude was quickly vanishing.

I was surprised to learn how chemotherapy treatments are administered. My preconceived ideas about it were along the lines of crawling into a big oven and a technician turning on the oven and baking me! But chemotherapy is nothing like that at all. In a large room at the hospital, there are two rows of lazy boy type reclining chairs.

This is the chemo room. I reported there once a week, and sat comfortably in one of the chairs; first, the nurse draws blood from my arm and sends it to the lab to check my white blood cell count and several other levels of concern to the doctor. If my blood panel results indicate that my system is still healthy enough to continue, the nurse returns and hangs a bottle of clear liquid (chemotherapy) on the I. V. stand, and for about an hour it drips slowly into my arm.

Including my check-in time, my blood test and the chemo-drip; most of my treatments lasted about four hours. Four hours of sitting on an easy chair and watching television, would not be a bad morning, but the chemo makes one feel queasy. I had chemotherapy treatments once a week.

My radiation mask was a tensile object. The day they made it was the day I realized this was all for real; but I still did not realize what I was in for. Every weekday, Monday through Friday, the technician fastened my head in the mask and the mask to the table so I would be in exactly the correct position for the ray gun! Then he positioned a huge ray gun at the specified exact coordinates and microwaved my neck! I received ninety seconds on the right side, ninety seconds on my left side, and one minute on the front. It left my mouth, throat, and sinuses feeling dry, like dessert sand on a summer afternoon! It burned the inside and the outside of my throat; it dried out my tongue and sinuses, temporarily eliminating my taste buds! For nine solid weeks I received these treatments!

Radiation treatments affect each patient differently, determining factors include; the location of the patients cancer and the number of treatments prescribed. Patients with head and neck cancer are affected the most adversely. That is because both the human neck and the human tongue become nearly dysfunctional while receiving radiation treatments. If you have either head or neck cancer, I would guess seventy five percent of your discomfort comes from your neck, throat and tongue. Take heart, the amazing products described in chapter

four will relieve most of your discomfort.

Chapter Four

That Knowing Smile

Your doctors are curing your cancer, they know that cancer left unchecked kills people; and they are saving your life; and they see many patients each month so they save many lives. Consequently, the burns you get from radiation, or the pimples from the chemotherapy, even the vomiting, hair loss and dry mouth are a small price to pay for good health. Your doctor knows these side effects are temporary and you will eventually recover from them.

They are considered small sacrifices for the life saving benefits you are receiving.

Many of these doctors have been specialist for years; they have seen many patients come and go. They know the treatments of today are both more effective and less painful than the treatments of twenty years ago. So, I would be surprised if your doctors were overly concerned with your suffering caused by the side effects. As the years have passed your doctor probably has developed two skills, one is to administer your cancer treatments, and the other is to ignore the temporary suffering it causes while it attacks your cancer.

My doctors advised me to tell them of every side effect caused by the treatments, and I did at first, fully expecting him to give me some advice or some prescription to help me feel better. But instead, I received a very consistent reaction from every medical professional I approached. I would report my side effects to them.

"It is hard to swallow, and I have a rash on my chest."

Instead of a prescription I always got the same reaction, an all-knowing smile would creep onto their faces and they would say one of the four following responses,

"Well, that just means the treatments are working." (I love a good sense of humor; but..)

"It will get much worse as we continue with your treatments." (Gee, thanks!)

"I know it's painful, but you will thank me later." (Is all that pain really necessary?)

"Well, in order to kill the cancer cells, we have to kill some healthy ones to." (Ouch!)

The medical professional's reactions were polished like diamonds and they stabbed at a patient. The reaction was typical of all of my doctors and nurses, because they had seen it all before, done it all before, and they knew how the routine usually went. Right about then, I began to take umbrage; my opinion and theirs was not exactly simpatico anymore; I consider myself a canny parson, and I apprised them that I was not going to take it anymore. Remember this, they are there to treat your cancer; not your side effects, you have to take your own initiative for relieving pain caused by treatments. The next chapter describes the specific, and near miraculous steps I took.

Chapter Five

Amazing Products

When a person is in a real crisis; the ability to take a tentative two and a problematic three and come up with the sum of a solid five is an invaluable trait!

These products relieved my neck from the terrible condition shown in the first three photo's below; and eventually completely healed it....*while I was still receiving chemotherapy and radiation treatments!* Note the beginning of healing in the fourth photo; and then nearly completely healed in the fifth photo….all the while still receiving daily radiation treatments! Amazing results! I shared these products with many of the other patients I saw every day at the treatment center and . . . they also, experienced phenomenal relief!

You might think you're a tough guy, and you don't need any relief from treatments because, hey the pain is only temporary, right? But, as you check out the pictures of me, you gotta ask yourself, are you ready to go through this? I'm sorry they are so graphic, and rest assured I'm okay now, so there is a happy ending here. The products in this book will practically eliminate these painful side effects, and still allow the cancer treatments to kill the cancer cells. (I am in full remission) Note the beginning of the healing process in pictures 4,5, and 6—important to realize, I was still receiving the treatments while I healed!

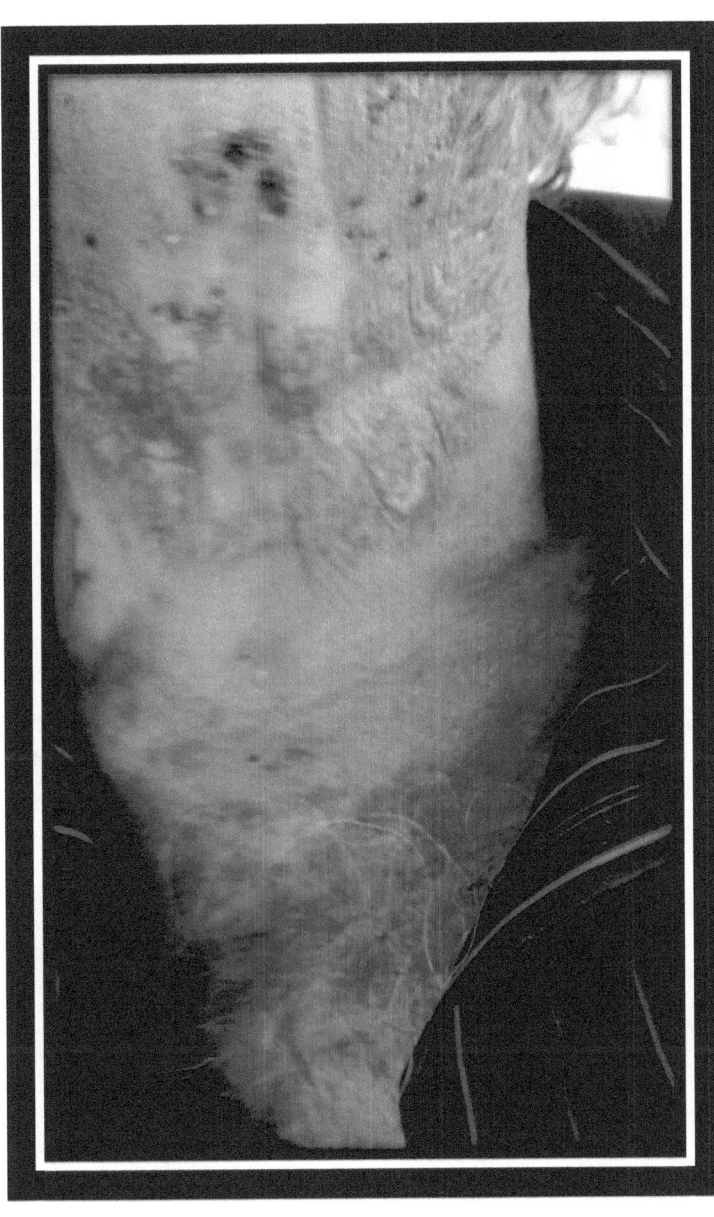

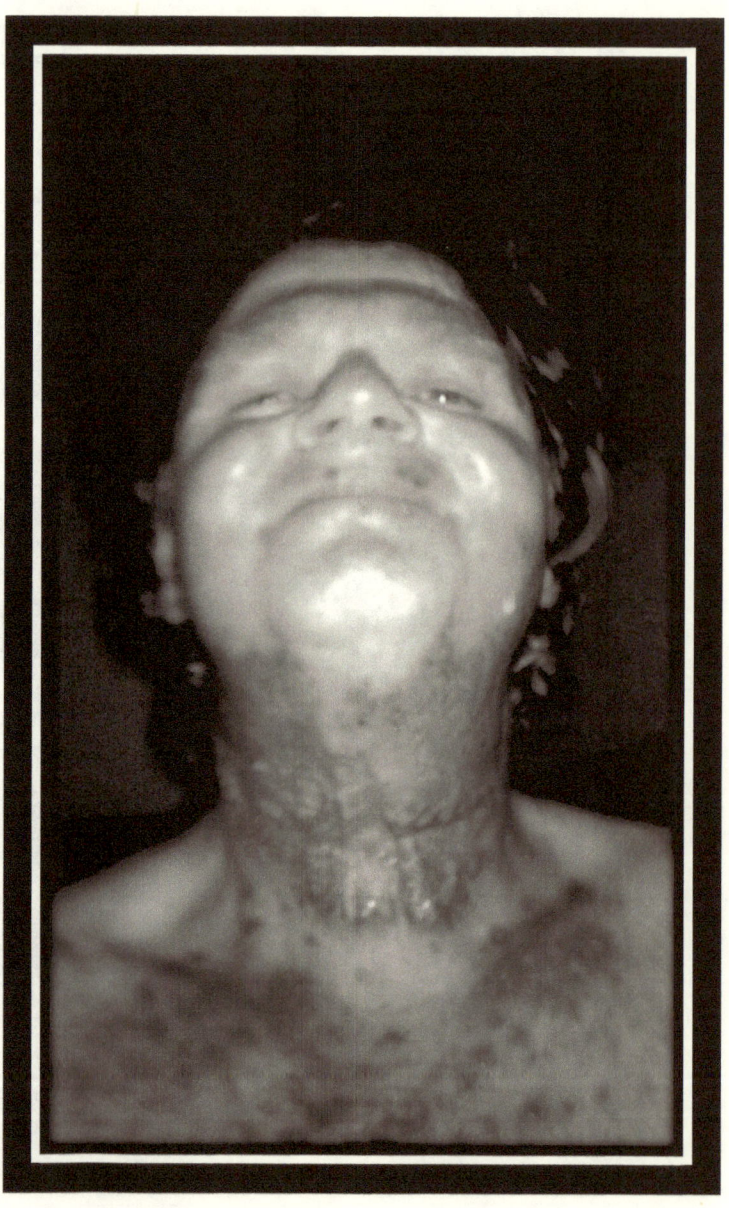

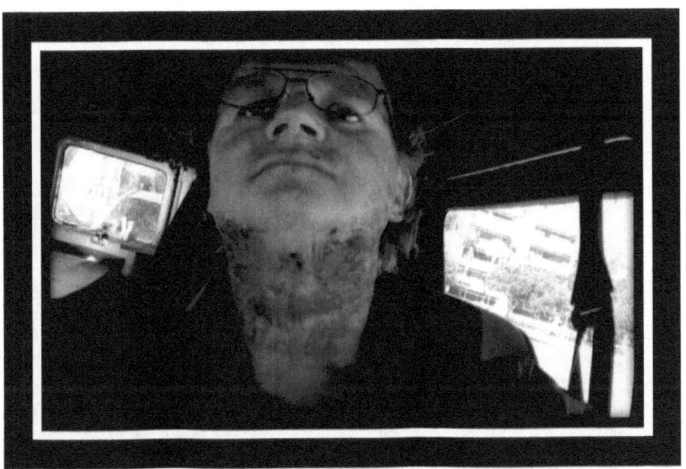

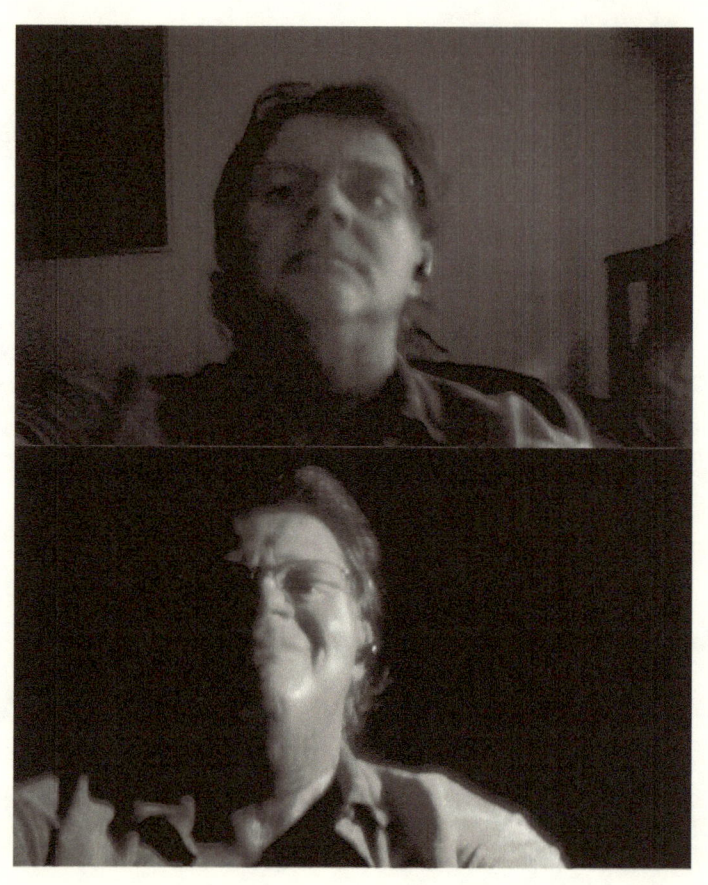

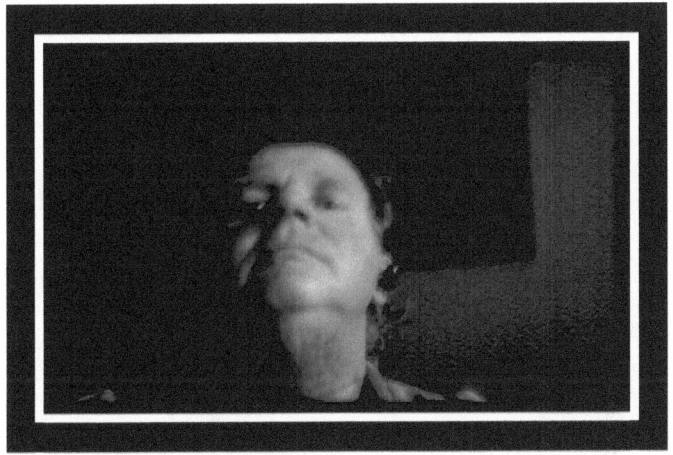

1. Iodex Ointment. This ointment is amazing in preventing or healing burns caused from radiation. Most pharmacies can get it for you in one day. Make sure to get the original formula, not scented and not the kind that heats up, as they will

cause irritation and stinging on your burned area. The original formula is the best. I recommend taking it off the radiation area before treatments; give the radiologist a clean, dry area to treat, but immediately after treatment, put this ointment on the entire area. It seems to stay on the skin quite a while; I usually applied it right after treatments, again right before bed, and again in the morning. My treatments were at 1:00 in the afternoon.

2. Olive Oil. My radiation treatments were on my neck. The bad news is, they are burning the inside just as badly as the outside, as made evident by the many patients who eventually need feeding tubes and cannot talk. I took three tablespoons of Olive oil every day; morning, noon, and night. I also recommend getting a good eye dropper and dropping some oil into your nose to relieve those dried out sinuses. When I did this, I could actually feel the relief in my sinuses.

3. Egg Whites. The human tongue was clearly not meant to handle radiation. I made a bad situation worse by trying to drink fresh citrus juice. NOT a good idea. My tongue seemed to develop a symmetrically perfect tic-tac-toe pattern of pimples on it. When I asked my doctor, she informed me that those were not pimples; they were my taste buds. Ouch! They hurt me more than any other side effect. The healing factor for my tongue was egg whites. I could not dream of

using a brush on my tender tongue, so I used my finger or just put the egg whites in my mouth and swished it around, I also drank a small amount for the benefit of my throat; remember I didn't start these treatments until after I was totally burned and could not swallow or talk anymore. Olive oil and egg whites healed my neck while I continued my treatments! So, after three weeks I was badly burned and could not swallow solid food; yet by my eighth and final week, I was seventy five per cent cured! An hour after swishing egg whites around my mouth, I would rinse with the salt and baking soda water solution (listed next) and my tongue healed completely while still receiving radiation treatments!

4. Salt and Baking Soda Water. Most of the things I ate or drank caused my tongue to sting. Chocolate flavored Ensure for instance, although vanilla Ensure did not. Whenever something made my tongue sting, I'd immediately

rinse with a salt and baking soda water solution. One-quarter cup of each per gallon of water. This probably contributed to healing my tongue, along with the egg whites, although I thought of the egg whites more as a healing treatment and this as a pain reliever. I found that by rinsing once or twice, my whole mouth, including my tongue, would be comfortable for an hour or two.

5. Electric Aloe is a powered mix that makes a lemonade type of drink. The company that makes it is called

Body Wise. You can try other means of hydration but this product will do the job like nothing else I've tried. Staying hydrated during your treatments can be a full time concern for some patients. This product is so effective I never had dry mouth once, even during treatments! I drank between two and four leaders a day. You can get it from a Body Wise dealer on the internet.

6. L-arginine Plus is a health product that is sold on the internet. It list

several health benefits such as; lowering blood pressure, promoting healthy heart health, helping to cleanse veins and arteries, and several others. I drank two quarts of it every day during my treatments for one reason, it refurbishes your body with nitrous oxide, and with my throat sore, I was not eating a regular diet. I really felt this product kept my strength up and my mood stable because my energy remained high for the full eight weeks of my treatments.

7. Preparation H on your face? I know it sounds odd, but it works for this. The type of chemotherapy I had was not standard chemotherapy. Many patients with head and neck cancer nowadays will get a more advanced form of chemotherapy, as I did. In place of traditional chemotherapy. It causes pimples on your face and neck. Well, they are not really pimples, I am told, but they are convincing imposters because they sure look like pimples. I tried putting many

creams on them, and one night, out of total desperation I remembered an ex-girlfriend of mine put preparation H on her face as a beauty cream! So, I put it on half of my face, and an antibody cream on the other half, I had at least 40 pimples on my face, so I put a it on thick. In the morning, the half with the Preparation H was very red, but the pimples were gone! The redness left in a day or two, and I found that using it very sparingly kept the pimples from returning, and did not cause such redness.

8. Protein Jell-O, ice Cream and Greek yogurt! Did anyone mention to you your diet is going to be limited during treatments? My throat was the worst during the third and fourth week; as I didn't use any of these products until after things became nearly intolerable. (about 4 and one-half weeks) But the two foods that I could always swallow and eat easily were Jell-O; and ice cream and yogurt mixed. So

I mixed some protein power in the Jell-O while making it, as your body needs protein every day and swallowing chunks of meat can be quite painful during treatments. Likewise, buy yogurt with protein in it and mix it with ice cream. You'll be losing weight anyway, and this ice cream treat provides your body with much of what it needs and is easy to get down. During my most trying weeks, all I ate was Jell-O with protein and ice cream mixed with yogurt. I drank a minimum of two quarts of Electric Aloe and two quarts of L-arginine every day; through my ten weeks of treatments, I never vomited, not even once! (In all honesty, about six different days, I had what I would call 'dry heaves' for about five minutes, but no food or liquid ever came up.) Sorry for the graphic report!

9. Vitamin Supplements are in season. I'm not going to debate if vitamins are good for us in our daily lives; but while you are receiving

treatments your body is under attack and needs all the support you can give it. I recommend an immune boost and a good multi vitamin at least; bear in mind you may prefer a liquid as opposed to a pill, which may be hard to swallow as the treatments progress.

10. Epson salts should be used early and often. Chemotherapy can cause your toe nails and finger nails to develop hang nail like sores; and if it spreads to six fingers and seven toes, it can be quite painful and

disabling. Start early with this, you will not be sorry, soak your feet and hands in warm water with Epson salt mixed in before you even get the first 'hang nail'. After you get one, continue soaking all of them, and when finished, put some Iodex ointment on the infected digit and wrap it up for several hours. This side effect is quite painful and if you control it early, you can save yourself unnecessary pain. These things are tough to get rid of once they get a toe hold, (so to speak, ha ha) so preventing them is advisable, however. If you do get infected by them, the treatment is the same; warm water, Epson Salt and Iodex Ointment in a wrap for several hours.

11. Ensure, for sure. Ensure is a healthy, nitrous drink that provides several basic dietary necessities. It is a liquid, so it is easy to get down. When my tongue was its worst, the chocolate flavor burned my tongue, but the vanilla flavor never did. Each serving provides about 350

calories, is easy to swallow, and helps keep your energy balanced during treatments.

12. Sleeping pills. I had a hard time sleeping during my ten weeks. In my discussions with other patients I learned that this was a common symptom. It may be because of all the pain, i.e. sore throat, tongue, and so on, or it may be the coughing that seemed to start the moment I laid down, either way, I found what worked the best for me was a combination pain killer and

sleeping pill. Tylenol PM, for example. Getting a decent night's sleep is essential. Remember this is only temporary, your body is trying to stay balanced, regulated and strong; but it needs your help in many ways. Regular sleep, a good hydration drink, and proper nutrition are three ways you can help your body to remain balanced.

13. Alternative Medication for Cancer. I remember the first morning after my surgical biopsy my doctor came

and told me the bad news; I had cancer, and it was not curable. But the next sentence he said was,

"Seek alternative healing, they can cure it, but we cannot!"

So, I followed my doctor's orders and after finishing chemotherapy and radiation treatments, I did some research, and the two companies I that impressed me the most with supplements that promote optimal health.. These companies' representatives made it very clear that these products do not cure anything and are not allowed to claim they do. So, I must change my terminology to clarify. These products help your body's cells in a way that promotes optimal health.

The first company is FKC, (friendship, kindness, and care) and they sell three products that are recommended for optimal health. Liver Right, Tri-antioxidant, and Ingenium.

The second company is Mannatach and one of their products is called

Ambrose. This product will also promote healthy cells and cell communication. Both of these companies can be found on the internet.

Anything Else You Can Think of;

Keep Thinking! I don't have all the answers, nor do I pretend that I do. The products I mentioned really helped me get through some tough treatments with some dignity and style. I had eight weeks of Chemo and 44 radiation treatments on my neck! As I mentioned, I was in very bad shape before I started helping myself. If you are scheduled for treatments, I urge you to take the side effects seriously and prevent as much discomfort as possible by starting to use these products in conjunction with your first scheduled treatment. Remember the truth is, you need the treatments, not the side effects.

Chapter Six

A Toast---

Here's to Remission!

Remission is the sweetest word a cancer patient will ever hear. Hopefully, by following doctor's orders, keeping your attitude positive, and staying hydrated, well-nourished, and getting regular sleep you have finished your treatments in fine style and you finally go on a follow up appointment and hear that sweetest of words; remission!

But what should you do now? I realize none of us can change our lives overnight, still it is nice to know which direction you should be heading. Lean muscle is the state of being your body should be gravitating towards. So, take some steps you're comfortable with to be sure you're getting the proper exercise. I realize it is tough to motivate yourself and make plans immediately following your treatments. However, there are several advantages to getting started right away; one advantage is you probably lost a few pounds while undergoing your treatments, so starting proper diet and exercise before you gain all that weight back makes sense, right? Most importantly, we need to form healthy living habits as soon as possible.

You don't have to make any changes! No one can force you to change and I know many cancer patients that go right back to their old habits after treatments. While receiving chemotherapy and radiation treatments; I saw one of my fellow patients outside smoking a cigarette, really? Is that how you want to play this hand? I am the kind of person that likes to give myself the best odds possible. If you really want to give yourself the best shot at a great life and keeping cancer in remission, make the changes you need to make. Ask your doctor about diet, exercise, smoking and drinking. I also recommend that you ask your doctor about the food supplements I recommended; but first, order a bottle and take the bottle to your doctor and let him evaluate it. Most doctors will say something like,

"It can't hurt anything." Hey, that's enough for me, if it can't hurt anything, and might do a world of good, and has helped some other people, why not take it. Some doctors are more encouraging about alternative medicines than others. Remember this, doctors are well educated, smart people, but they are human. So if your doctor doesn't do backflips when you show him food supplements that may help you, don't sweat it; if he says it won't interfere with whatever he is giving you, and it won't hurt to take them, consider that to be his blessing of approval and proceed. Never allow a doctors lack of enthusiasm for an alternative cure affect your decision to use it. Do your own research, make up your own mind, I recommend clearing it with your doctor, then move forward with it; it may save your life!

If you need to make dietary changes, now is the time. Eliminating unhealthy habits should be a top priority for you now as well. You can achieve 'lean' by diet alone; but to achieve *lean muscles* you will need to exercise regularly.

Just hearing the word 'cancer' freaks many people out so I want to encourage you not to react with consternation. Don't worry if some of your friends and family are uncertain around you when they first hear the news. Give them time to see your strengths and weaknesses, and stay cheerful; consider the cancer an imp in your life, don't work yourself into frenzy by imagining the worse possible results. Once people see you going on with your life, dealing with your cancer like it is an enigma, yet maintaining a state of repose, they will figure it all out. Be patient, they will adjust proportionately to how you adjust, so as much as possible, take it all in stride, never missing a step, and oh yea, good luck with that! You'll have your moments of doubt, but publically I recommend that you remain pragmatic, optimistic and canny! There is no point to invoking others pity; besides your strength will pique their curiosity!

Chapter Seven

Aftermath:

Continuing ....

with the Healing Process

It's not over when the treatments are finished; el facto, many patients consider this to be the time of the greatest discomfort! Personally, I was beat down to a frazzle! Whipped like a tired dog. The

44 radiation treatments I had was more than any other patients in our gaggle received. The eight weeks of chemo was also the longest stint of our group. I was exhausted from it all. I held up strong and steady through the whole series of treatments, but I was surprised at how exhausted I was at the end. It was time to re-group.

First things first, it may seem contradictory but the best way to rebuild your energy level is to eat fairly light, engage in light exercise regularly, shower and bathe regularly, and sleep a lot.

Besides a lot of sleep, resting also is important; all that seems obvious, right? But doing all that was very tough for me the first month. Luckily for me my neck sores were healed completely by time I finished treatments, so, I could eat soft food, I could drink liquids and I could sleep comfortably; but I still could not speak, and my energy level was so low, I could barely get out of bed!

    I had lost my voice completely during the first four weeks of treatments, and although the healing products I used healed many other side-effects completely, my voice took about three weeks after all the treatments were finished to return to me.

But for that first month following my treatments I forced myself to get out of bed about eight or nine o'clock, do five push-ups with my hands on the table and my feet on the floor, then do five half squats, then shower, drink a breakfast shake and then go back to bed and watch a movie. Most days I fell back asleep because that little bit of activity exhausted me. At twelve noon or one o'clock I'd wake up and do it all again; and then once more in the evening. I remember thinking showering three times a day was a huge amount of activity, but something about the cool water refreshed me, even if only for a few minutes.

But I'm a go getter, I was not used to being that tired, and my exhausted state of being upset me greatly; I found a good product that helped me get some of my energy back. It is called EMERGE and it is available through a company called Max Muscle. You can find them online at; *www.maxmuscle.com* I prefer the Wild Cherry Tart flavor. Use as directed, more to come later about that product. I did not know for sure if I would ever feel enlivened again. But let me assure you, after the month passed, I had 75 % of my pre-cancer treatment energy back, and a year later I had probably 90% of my old schedule back; I don't believe to this day I'm one hundred percent and may never be again, but I'm okay with where I am now.

    I guess my point is this; I know how tired you feel, but get up and get the blood flowing several times a day; and take your vitamins and drink your shakes and eat what you can. Shower or bathe, using the water will refresh and restore, eventually. By doing that rather than just lying in bed waiting for your strength to return, I believe you can shorten your recovery time considerably.

It is apropos to discuss dry mouth; thee one symptom my doctors assured me would be with me for life. Since my glands were burned by radiation, my body has no way to make saliva; you may have heard this already. Well, I make no promises, but last month I felt it for the first time, the miracle of saliva wetting my mouth again! I have had a total of three such occurrences so far since my cancer treatments.

There are very few times in my life I have used the expression, I'd sell my soul for this or that. But after one lives with dry mouth for a while, you want it to end pretty badly, at least I did.

I have no magic cures, but I will share seven nouns that you may eventually consider magical words if you get the same results I have gotten. Peppermint tea; Biotene oral spray; olive oil; and one adjective and one verb that makes the whole plan work; hot and fasting. (I also put one tea spoon of Emerge in each pot of my tea, it may or may help with my dry mouth, but it does boost my energy)

    Here is how it worked for me; because of my dry mouth, I quit drinking plain water because it was just ineffective. I tentatively tried drinking many other liquids; first I tried a olive oil mixture, but the first one I made was too oily. I learned an oily mouth was not as good as one containing nature's saliva, yet it was better than one that felt a dry as dessert sand! Still, I grew weary of my mouth always feeling oily.

One day, I discovered a decent drink that was not so oily. I have used it every day since, it's a simple recipe really; I made some peppermint tea, I added about a teaspoon of olive oil to a one liter bottle, and a couple squirts of Biotene Oral Spray, (available at most drugstores and Walmart) and I added a tea spoon of Emerge energy drink and the result was a drink that was very satisfying to me. I have since made it with peach tea and enjoy that sometimes for a change. I must also mention that I sometimes drink it chilled and sometimes drink it hot; on all three days that I experienced the return of some salvia, I was drinking hot tea all day. I usually drink about four liters a day because it is all I drink. But this was a big improvement for me, because water did not quench my dry mouth, I had often had drank a full case, (16 liters) in a single day. My doctor told me that was too much liquid, and that I was working my kidneys too hard, so I was happy for the relief the tea provided.

Also because of my spiritual beliefs, I fast occasionally. I simply spend one day not eating anything at all, but instead drinking protein drinks and whatever else I want to drink. The reason I bring this up is because all three times I have felt salvia in my mouth, I had not eaten all day; I usually had drank about six liters of the peppermint tea mixture, and viola… there it was… good old fashion saliva in my mouth, the kind I can spit with! It has been about a year since my last treatment. I'm hopeful that this healing trend will continue. Dry mouth is very inconvenient.

I still have dry mouth often; I still drink my tea mixture; for me, that has been the best compromise. But a few days of salvia incidents promoted hope in my heart of hearts; perhaps one day, we both will be free from dry mouth! It is as if a demon has stolen one of our keys; but perhaps we can find another!

Chapter Eight

The- -Why Me?- - Thing

Nine out of ten people think a rose is a pretty flower; they think mashed potatoes and gravy is tasty enough to eat; and nine out of ten cancer patients wonder, why me?

If you are that special tenth person that does not wonder; I may give you an askance, but this chapter is not dutiful reading for you. To the other nine who do wonder, for what it is worth, here is my insight on the topic.

The meaning of life can be described accurately many different ways. A pastor may say we are here to learn to love one another; while a judge may feel mankind was put here to learn justice, order and discipline. Far be it for me to feel qualified to argue with anyone's take on the meaning of life. I am sure there are many accurate descriptions; the specific area I'd like to examine now is this; is part of life a series of test?

    I believe it is; it may not be the ultimate meaning of life, yet I will always believe it is a part of why we are here. Earth is many things to many people, but I believe it is a testing ground for every human that was ever born here!
The rich and the poor are tested, the famous and the infamous, males and females, every race, every religion, everyone is tested here is some way.

Any cancer patient can react with consternation and push themselves into a frenzy trying to figure out if you have somehow merited this disease or if it just per chance dropped in on you. You will find your answer if you befriend the other cancer patients you encounter. You will find that some smoked, but many did not; some are admitted sinners, but many seen almost saintly. Some are rude and unfriendly, but many are very nice and very friendly; some have a family history of cancer, but then again many do not. Some are Christians, but some are not. In fact the one thing all these people have in common is this; they all have cancer! Some are young, some older; some are men, some are women.

So, as you can see, who cancer attacks is an enigma. Some day we all may know more. But for today, my gaggle of cancer friends and I agreed on this; no matter if you are a man, woman or child; of any race or religion; rich or poor; a savant or uneducated……….. Cancer will test you; cancer treatments will test your resolve!

I apologize if the simplicity of my philosophy does not cover it all for you. I cannot explain the whole of it because no one can yet, we will eventually learn more about it, I am sure, but until that time; consider it a test of sorts, a trial by fire, so to speak. One woman said, God wanted my attention and when my body was attacked, my spirit began to roar!

I cannot explain to you why you got cancer, in fact, I feel the question is nearly a paradox. Smoking does cause it in some people but not others! Why? Even in families more prone to it, certain members are unaffected! Why? And on and on; no one knows those answers yet, so why beat yourself up over this unanswerable enigma?

Perhaps the better questions are; what can I do to promote optimal health in my future? Can I help other cancer patients in any way? Can I find the courage to continue planning my future? Why do you have cancer? The very question intrudes into the imagination and exist only as a paradox!

My final analysis, for what it is worth is this; allow yourself to consider this a test of your resolve that fate itself bestowed upon you. Then set out to pass this test! This is a time for you to shine; make _all_ the right moves, _all_ the right choices, and make every attempt to step through this hoop with grace and dignity. Muster your effrontery; refuse to be beset by this cancer test! Be a good patient, do your own research, find your own solutions and follow through with the best plan you can conceive to return yourself to optimal health and a normal future!

 Having said that, it is time for me to close. I wish you the very best of good fortune. May every prayer you invoke be answered to your favor, and may you win your battle with this contemptible disease. I cannot fight your battle for you, no one can fight this battle for you; I am willingly giving you my support, my advice and my story; now it is up to you, go fight your battle!

Questions? Comments? Suggestions?

E-mail author Chase Kennedy at:

hurkmebaby@yahoo.com

Other books written by Chase Kennedy

(available at Amazon Books)

Unjustly Accused! is based on a true story about a woman accused of killing her husband and her three sons! Set in Michigan around the turn of the century, this story holds such intrigue that a Hollywood producer contacted me about turning it into a movie! After a year of discussion, it is finally being turned into a script! So, I'm keeping my hopes alive that it will soon be a movie; but either way, it is an exciting and factual read with many good reviews!

Me and Jesus Homeless in Burbank! It is not just a spiritual story; it is an entertaining story that really packs a wallop! It is over four hundred pages long and as deep as the ocean! *Me and Jesus Homeless in Burbank*! has been voted:

The most enlightening spiritual book of the year; by Avid Book Club readers! The books 426 pages present a quintessential human story of a man who meets an extraordinary spiritual friend. Spiritually enlightening and biblically correct, this book delivers the story of Christianity as never presented before! Partial to neither denominations nor ancestry, *Me and Jesus Homeless in Burbank!* explains many of the <u>whys</u> and <u>how's</u> of the bible while the story itself keeps readers entertained! One reader called it: *Tomato Sweet!*

A special group of people were chosen to test read this book before it was released; the results were more than I ever could have expected! After reading this book, all of them said the storyline was heartfelt and interesting throughout the entire 426 pages! They also said they felt they understood the bible better, and they felt closer to Jesus, and they were now certain they were children of God. Many of them said they felt sadness when they reached the end of the story!

If you already are a Christian, I hope this book renews and refreshes your beliefs and your faith. If you haven't made that leap into Christianity yet, I hope reading this story causes you to reflect on what that decision could mean in your life; but I also hope the plot intrigue's and entertains you! The title was carefully chosen to pique your interest; while at the same time accurately alludes at the facts of the story effrontery. This book took me literally years to write, and I am proud of it; I hope you will apprize it, as I do. I believe this book is so vibrant, spiritual, and alive; it could change people's lives!

Loving the Addicted Beyond Their Addictions! is tentatively scheduled for release on October 15th, 2012. Since it has not been released yet, there are no reviews, but I feel it is up to the same standard as my other books. I always strive for interesting storylines that have some root in a true story, a good character mix and it is also my intention to write books that are useful, books that inform, educate or at least are apposite to the points I am trying to share. This book should be in the hands of every parent (and other relatives) that have a loved one addicted to drugs or alcohol! It contains list of what to do, and what not to do. The story itself is subject to a kind of grueling realism that exists whenever dealing with an addict; but it is mixed with humor, interesting characters abound, and somehow this true story ended up with a happy ending! I believe it also will hold most readers interest; It steps up to the plate and delivers good, solid advice that a parent can put to use immediate use and perhaps help rescue a loved one from an addiction, before it is too late.

Last Chance Love - - - anticipated release date is 12/15/12

The Weight Loss Book for Men - - - anticipated release date is 12/15/12

Open Amazon Books and type Chase Kennedy in the search bar, all of my current books should be listed; both as paperbacks and on Amazon's kindle.

Chase Kennedy; A Short Biography:

I wasn't always a paper back writer, for many years, I was a news and sports reporter. Many times I had to write my own stories and report information live! Eventually I noticed my writing was getting more accolades than my reporting. Eventually the inevitable came to pass, my reporting career ended and writing became my solo career!

www.ingramcontent.com/pod-product-compliance
Lightning Source LLC
Chambersburg PA
CBHW030817180526
45163CB00003B/1321